HEALING
HASHIMOTO'S
THYROID
COOKBOOK

**SIMPLE AND EFFECTIVE RECIPES TO HELP RELIEVE
THE SYMPTOMS OF HASHIMOTO'S THYROIDITIS**

 CookNation

HEALING HASHIMOTO'S THYROID COOKBOOK

SIMPLE AND EFFECTIVE RECIPES TO HELP RELIEVE THE SYMPTOMS OF HASHIMOTO'S THYROIDITIS

ISBN: 978-1-912511-94-5

DISCLAIMER

CONTENTS

DINNER RECIPES

DESSERT & SNACK RECIPES

INTRODUCTION

Discovering that you suffer from thyroid disease can be a challenge which requires lifestyle changes, including learning how to adapt your diet. A healthy, nutritious way of eating can complement other treatments that you may be receiving and help alleviate symptoms, as well as making you fitter, healthier and stronger.

WHAT IS HASHIMOTO'S DISEASE?

Hashimoto's is the most common form of thyroiditis, or inflammation of the thyroid gland. It is an autoimmune disease which leads to the body attacking the thyroid gland: a small butterfly shaped gland in the neck which produces the hormones that regulate and control your body's growth and metabolism.

Hashimoto's, named after Japanese physician Hakaru Hashimoto who published the first description of the condition in 1912, is a progressive disease that develops very slowly, therefore sufferers may have had it for many years before developing symptoms and receiving a diagnosis.

SYMPTOMS

As the thyroid gland is destroyed over time, it becomes less able to produce the thyroid hormone and sufferers will begin to experience symptoms of hypothyroidism (otherwise known as an underactive thyroid). The most common initial symptoms are tiredness, weight gain, dry skin or a lump in the throat known as a goiter. It is also possible that suffers may experience:

· Increased sensitivity to cold
· Constipation
· A puffy face
· Brittle nails
· Hair loss
· Enlargement of the tongue
· Muscle aches, tenderness and stiffness
· Joint pain and stiffness
· Muscle weakness
· Excessive or prolonged menstrual bleeding (menorrhagia)
· Depression
· Memory lapses

If you are experiencing these symptoms you should consult a physician.

DIAGNOSIS

If your doctor suspects that you may suffer from an underactive thyroid, they are likely to perform a blood test to measure the levels of thyroid hormone and thyroid-stimulating hormone (TSH) produced by your pituitary gland (a tiny organ found at the base of the brain).

If you test positively for thyroid disease, then you will most likely have this same test regularly to ensure that your hormone levels are under control and that your medication is working correctly. Initially this may be frequent, but once your symptoms are under control it's likely to reduce to once a year.

CAUSES

The causes of Hashimoto's disease and this is the reason some people's bodies attack their immune system is unknown, while there are different theories; some scientists think a virus or bacterium might trigger your immune system to begin attacking itself, but others believe a genetic flaw may be involved. Either way, the main cause of the disease is yet to be discovered. There are, however, risk factors that make it more likely that you will be a sufferer. These can include:

- Gender: Women are much more likely than men to develop Hashimoto's disease.
- Age: Hashimoto's disease can occur at any age but must commonly occurs between the ages of 30 and 50.
- Hereditary factors: You're at higher risk for Hashimoto's disease if other family members have thyroid or other autoimmune diseases.
- Other autoimmune diseases: Having another autoimmune disease, such as rheumatoid arthritis, type 1 diabetes or lupus, increases your risk of developing an underactive thyroid.
- Radiation exposure: People exposed to excessive levels of environmental radiation are more prone to Hashimoto's disease than those who have never suffered from exposure.
- Excessive iodine: Research suggests certain drugs and too much iodine, a trace element required by your body to make thyroid hormones, may trigger thyroid disease in susceptible people. This is slightly controversial however, and a diet which contains iodine is necessary for good management of the illness.

TREATMENT

Unfortunately, there is no cure for Hashimoto's disease, but there are a variety of treatment options that you can explore with your doctor.

Generally, treatment involves taking artificially created hormones to restore your metabolism and regulate your hormone levels. The most commonly used medication is levothyroxine, a thyroid hormone replacement medication, and it is usually taken for life.

DIET

In addition to prescribed medication, a healthy diet can help regulate your hormone levels and keep the symptoms of thyroid disease under control. There are many different diets that can be used to help alleviate symptoms and it is likely that a degree of experimentation will be required to find what works best for you. Below you will find outlined the most commonly used diets to help you manage your health and feel nourished.

ELIMINATION DIET

Many sufferers of Hashimoto's disease experience food intolerances and elimination diets are a good way of establishing if you are one of them. In order to do this, for three weeks you should exclude the following common food allergens:

- Alcohol
- Gluten
- Dairy
- Soy
- Eggs
- Corn
- Nuts
- Shellfish
- Preservatives

You MUST be strict in ensuring that all food you consume during this three week period does not contain any of the above as it will skew your results. At the end of the three week period you should gradually reintroduce the foods, one every four days, in the following order:

- Eggs
- Nuts
- Shellfish
- Corn
- Preservatives
- Soy
- Dairy
- Gluten

You should keep a keen eye on any symptoms you experience whilst re-introducing the foods, note them down and stop consuming them if you get an adverse reaction. You should then continue to reintroduce the foods in the order stated above.

OTHER DIETS

Some people may not wish, or be unable, to commit to an elimination diet. If this is the case, then research has shown that people who suffer from Hasmimoto's disease may also benefit from a gluten-free diet, as the most common food sensitivity for people suffering from Hashimoto's is gluten.

However, unless you suffer from celiac disease, or have found that you have a sensitivity by following the elimination diet, it is not necessary to exclude all gluten (which is a protein found in wheat, barley, rye, and other grains) from your diet.

It is beneficial for many to exclude pasta, bread, baked goods, beer, and cereals and instead focus on foods that are naturally gluten-free, such as vegetables, fruits, lean meats, seafood, beans, legumes, nuts, and eggs.

A paleo or autoimmune modified paleo diet

A paleo diet seeks to mimic the diet of our earliest ancestors and followers eat unprocessed, naturally occurring foods such as; meat, vegetables, nuts, seeds, seafood, and healthy fats, including avocado and olive oil. It excludes the consumption of grains, dairy, potatoes, beans, lentils, refined sugar, and refined oils.

An autoimmune paleo diet (AIP) follows these principles, but also excludes nightshade vegetables (such as tomatoes, eggplant, bell peppers, cayenne pepper and paprika), eggs, nuts, and seeds. This is because these foods can trigger inflammation and a flare up of symptoms in sufferers of a variety of autoimmune diseases.

A low glycaemic index diet

A low glycaemic index, or low-GI, diet involves eating foods that are low on the glycaemic index, a scale that indicates the effect of a particular food on a person's blood sugar levels.
Eating foods that are low-GI help people have more stable blood sugar levels, causing them to feel fuller for longer and experience fewer hormone fluctuations. This diet has also been found to help people with type-2 diabetes , as well as lowering the risk of heart disease.

People with Hasmimoto's benefit from eating nutritionally dense food that helps support the struggling immune system. The following nutrients are essential to ensuring thyroid health:

· Iodine – found in seafood, table salt, dairy products, eggs and prunes
· Selenium- found in eggs, pork, Brazil nuts, tuna, sardines, beef and chicken
· Zinc- found in shellfish, beef, chicken, legumes such as lentils, beans and cow's milk

The recipes in this book are all designed to help your body heal and, therefore assist in relieving symptoms of hypothyroidism. As such, they are all made with unprocessed food, healthy fats, no refined carbohydrates or sugars and limited nightshade vegetables. They also contain healthy levels of iodine, selenium and zinc.

They focus on using vegetables, fruits, lean meats and nuts, and are low-GI, which will help you feel full and satisfied, as well as healthy. This book is not a substitute for medical advice however, and is to be used in conjunction with your physician's directions. Many thyroid medications require that you don't eat for two hours before taking to ensure they're properly absorbed. Please check yours before indulging.

Following broad Hashimoto principles, the recipes in this collection are bursting with fresh, vibrant and delicious flavours. Improving your diet, health and lifestyle has never tasted so good!

BREAKFAST
RECIPES

TROPICAL BREAKFAST SMOOTHIE

Ingredients

- 1 tin of coconut milk
- 1 banana
- 75g/3oz fresh or frozen pineapple, chopped
- 45g/1½oz fresh or frozen mango
- 1 tbsp protein powder (optional)

Method

1 Combine the coconut milk, banana, pineapple, mango and, if using, the protein powder in a blender and blitz on high until smooth.

2 Serve in a tall glass or travel mug if you're on the go.

CHEF'S NOTE

A smoothie is a great way to start the day when you're in a rush. This version is bursting with antioxidants and tastes like a piña colada. The coconut milk is packed full of healthy fats that will keep you full until lunchtime.

MIDDLE-EASTERN EGGS

Ingredients

- 1 tbsp olive oil
- 1 large onion, chopped
- 1 red and 1 green pepper, cut into long slices
- 1 garlic clove, crushed
- ½ tsp cumin powder
- ½ tsp cayenne pepper
- 1 tbsp tomato purée
- 4 salad tomatoes, chopped
- 4 eggs

To serve:
- 4 tbsp Greek yogurt

Method

1 Heat the olive oil in a large, lidded frying pan. Add the onions, peppers and garlic, then season with salt and pepper. Cook on a medium heat until soft. Add in the cumin and the cayenne pepper.

2 Stir in the tomato purée and cook for a couple more minutes, before adding the tomatoes with a splash of water.

3 Simmer for 10 minutes or so, uncovered, until reduced a little and the tomatoes are soft. If it becomes too thick (it should have a pasta sauce consistency) then add a touch more water.

4 Make 4 small wells in the sauce and break an egg into each. Place the lid on the pan and cook for roughly 4 mins or until the whites are just set and the yolks are still runny.

5 Serve with the yogurt drizzled on the top.

CHEF'S NOTE

These eggs are an unusual and tasty way to start the day and scale up brilliantly for a brunch with friends or family. The tomatoes and peppers make this unsuitable to anybody with sensitivity to nightshade vegetables.

FLOURLESS PANCAKES

Ingredients

- 1½ large ripe bananas
- 2 eggs
- ½ tsp vanilla extract
- ¼ tsp ground cinnamon
- 1/8 tsp baking powder

To serve:
- Fresh fruits
- Greek yogurt

Method

1 Crack the eggs in a bowl and lightly whisk, then mash the bananas with a potato masher or a fork in another bowl.

2 Add the egg, baking powder, vanilla and cinnamon to the bananas and stir to combine.

3 Heat a frying pan on a medium-low heat and pour about 2 tbsp of the batter into the pan to cook until the bottom appears set (1 to 2 minutes). Flip with a spatula and cook a further minute. Repeat until all of the batter is used.

4 Serve immediately, topped with fresh fruit and/or yogurt

CHEF'S NOTE

Everyone loves pancakes for a breakfast treat and this flourless version allows you to indulge, whilst maintaining a gluten-free start to the day.

APPLE PIE GRANOLA BITES

Ingredients

- 125g/4oz apple, grated
- 125g/4oz raw pecans
- 125g/4oz almonds
- 10 medjool dates, pitted

- 125g/4oz almond butter
- 125g/4oz coconut flakes
- ½ tsp ground cinnamon
- ½ tsp vanilla extract

Method

1 Pulse the pecans and almonds in a food processor until they reach a flour-like consistency then place them in a large bowl.

2 Process the dates in the food processor until they turn into a soft paste.

3 Add the date paste to the nuts and combine with all of the remaining ingredients, stirring until everything is well combined.

4 Divide the mixture into tablespoon-sized portions and squeeze together to form a ball.

5 Refrigerate for an hour or two and then serve.

CHEF'S NOTE

Perfect for food on the go, these breakfast bites are best made at the weekend, as they will happily keep in the fridge for a week, allowing you to grab one each morning.

BLUEBERRY MUFFINS

Ingredients

- 125g/4oz blanched almond flour
- Pinch of baking soda
- Pinch of salt
- 2 tbsp raw honey

- 120ml/4fl oz coconut milk
- 2 tbsp coconut oil, melted
- 1 egg
- 60g/2½ oz fresh blueberries

Method

1 Preheat the oven to 190C/350F/Gas mark 5 and line a muffin tin with paper cases or use a non-stick silicone muffin pan.

2 Mix together the almond flour, baking soda and salt.

3 In a separate bowl, whisk together the honey, coconut milk, coconut oil, and egg.

4 Mix the wet and dry ingredients together until just combined, but be careful not to over mix.

5 Gently fold in the blueberries into the batter.

6 Spoon batter into the prepared muffin tin, filling each to the top.

7 Bake for around 20-25 mins, until a skewer inserted into the centre comes out clean.

8 Wait until muffins are completely cool before serving.

CHEF'S NOTE
Experimenting with different types of gluten-free flours is a fantastic way to allow you to enjoy your favourite baked goods, which you may have thought were out of bounds.

SWEET POTATO WAFFLE

Ingredients

- 1 sweet potato, peeled and grated
- 1 large egg
- 2 tbsp coconut flour
- ½ tsp salt

Method

1 Preheat a waffle iron. Meanwhile, stir together the grated sweet potato, egg, coconut flour and salt.

2 Spray the waffle iron generously with non-stick spray.

3 Spoon half of the sweet potato mixture into the centre of the waffle iron. Close the lid and cook for 5-8 minutes, or until the waffle begins to turn a medium golden brown.

4 Remove the waffle and repeat with second half of the batter.

CHEF'S NOTE

This plant-based waffle also works perfectly as a pancake mix. Top with savoury guacamole and poached eggs, or make a sweet treat with agave syrup and fresh fruits.

BAKED AVOCADOS

Ingredients

- 1 avocado
- 2 eggs
- 2 slices of multiseed or rye bread

- 2 tsp flat-leaf parsley, chopped

Method

1 Preheat the oven to 180C/350F/Gas mark 4. Cut the avocado in half, remove the stone and scoop a little extra of the flesh out.

2 Break the first egg into a bowl. Using a spoon, place the yolk in half of the avocado, then carefully start to add the white (you may not manage to add it all). Season with salt and pepper, then repeat with the other egg and avocado half.

3 Place the avocado halves in a small baking dish that fits them snugly and bake for 15-20 minutes, or until the white is opaque and the yolk is cooked to your liking.

4 Toast the bread and serve with the avocado, seasoned with salt and pepper and a scattered with the parsley.

CHEF'S NOTE
A tasty alternative to avocado on toast, this dish looks and tastes great.

VANILLA BREAKFAST BOWL

Ingredients

- 50g/2oz jumbo porridge oats
- 200ml/7fl oz unsweetened almond milk
- ½ tsp vanilla extract
- 2 tbsp natural yogurt
- 25g/1oz chia seeds

Method

1 Mix all of the ingredients in a bowl and leave to soak for at least 20 mins.

2 Once the oats have softened if you find the porridge is too dry, add a little water.

3 Divide the mixture between 2 bowls and top each with blueberries, flaked almonds and honey, or any other combination of fruit and nuts you would prefer.

CHEF'S NOTE

A filling, low GI breakfast that will keep you full until lunchtime and can be made the night before. Why not try with raspberries and chopped hazelnuts?

VEGGIE BREAKFAST BAKE

Ingredients

- 2 large field mushrooms
- 4 tomatoes, halved
- 1 garlic clove, thinly sliced
- 2 tsp olive oil
- 200g/7oz bag of spinach
- 2 eggs

Method

1 Preheat the oven to 200C/400F/Gas 6. Put the mushrooms and tomatoes into an ovenproof dish, scatter over the garlic and drizzle over the oil with some seasoning, before baking for 10 mins.

2 Whilst the mushrooms and tomatoes are cooking, put the spinach into a large colander, then pour over a kettle of boiling water to wilt it. Squeeze out any excess water before adding the spinach to the dish.

3 Make 2 little gaps between the vegetables and crack the eggs into them. Return to the oven and cook for a further 8-10 mins or until the egg is cooked to your liking.

CHEF'S NOTE
This breakfast bake contains three of your five a day! Serve with chilli sauce to kick-start your day.

BOILED EGGS WITH MARMITE SOLDIERS

Ingredients

- 2 eggs
- 4 slices wholemeal bread
- A knob of butter
- Marmite
- Mixed seeds to serve

Method

1 Place the eggs in a saucepan of water and bring to the boil, Leave the eggs in boiling water for 3 mins and then remove.

2 Meanwhile, toast the bread and spread thinly with butter, then Marmite.

3 To serve, cut into soldiers, dip into the egg, then sprinkle a few mixed seeds on top.

CHEF'S NOTE
A good source of iodine and selenium, the Marmite and seeds put a new spin on a childhood classic of dippy eggs and soldiers.

GARLIC MUSHROOM FRITTATA

Ingredients

- 1 tbsp olive oil
- 250g/9oz sliced chestnut mushrooms
- 1 crushed garlic clove

- 1 tbsp thinly sliced fresh chives
- 4 large beaten eggs
- Freshly ground black pepper

Method

1 Heat the oil in a small frying pan over a high heat. Stir-fry the mushrooms in three batches for 2-3 mins, or until softened. Tip the cooked mushrooms into a sieve and drain the excess cooking juice.

2 Return all the mushrooms to the pan and stir in the garlic and chives with a pinch of ground black pepper. Cook for a further minute, then reduce the heat to low.

3 Preheat the grill to its hottest setting. Pour the eggs over the mushrooms. Cook for five mins, or until almost set.

4 Place the pan under the grill for 3-4 mins until set. Serve immediately, or allow to cool.

CHEF'S NOTE

Mushrooms and eggs are high in protein and make a quick, filling meal at any time of the day. This frittata would also be great as a lunch or light dinner, served with salad.

OVERNIGHT OATS

Ingredients

- 50g/1¾oz porridge oats
- 2 coarsely grated apples
- 20g/¾oz roughly chopped blanched hazelnuts
- ¼ tsp ground cinnamon

- ¼ tsp ground nutmeg
- 200g/7oz Greek yogurt
- 100ml/3½fl oz skimmed milk
- 100g/3½oz blueberries
- 2 tsp toasted, flaked almonds

Method

1 In a bowl mix the oats, apples, hazelnuts, cinnamon and nutmeg.

2 Stir in the yogurt and milk, cover the bowl before leaving the mixture to chill in the fridge for several hours, or overnight.

3 When ready to serve, spoon into two bowls and top with the blueberries and flaked almonds.

CHEF'S NOTE

High in protein and low on the GI scale, this is a great breakfast for weekday mornings as all of the prep can be done in advance, meaning that its just as easy as pouring out a bowl of cereal-but much healthier.

PUMPKIN-SPICE GRANOLA

Ingredients

- 225g/8oz unsweetened coconut flakes
- 75g/3oz raisins
- 75g/3oz chopped dried apple
- 2 medium ripe bananas
- 2 tbsp melted coconut oil

- 1 ½ tsp cinnamon
- 1 tsp ground ginger
- ½ tsp ground mace
- ¼ tsp sea salt

Method

1 Preheat your oven to 150C/300F/Gas 2 and line a baking sheet with parchment paper.

2 In a medium mixing bowl, stir together the coconut flakes, raisins and apple.

3 In a separate bowl, mash the banana until smooth, then stir in the coconut oil, spices, and sea salt.

4 Add the wet and dry mixtures together and stir until well combined and everything sticks together.

5 Spread out evenly onto the prepared baking sheet.

6 Bake for 45 to 50 mins, stirring halfway through, until the granola is a golden brown.

7 Leave to cool for at least 15 mins to set. Break any large chunks into smaller, bite-sized pieces.

CHEF'S NOTE

Granola is great to batch cook and have on the go for breakfast served with yogurt or milk. This version, if served with unsweetened nut milk, is suitable for those following an AIP or autoimmune diet.

CARROT CAKE SMOOTHIE

Ingredients

- 1 apple
- ½ large carrot
- 1 medium banana
- 1 cup of ice

- ½ tbsp coconut oil
- 120ml/4fl oz coconut milk
- Dash of cinnamon, nutmeg and cloves

Method

1 Core, peel and chop the apple.

2 Peel and chop the carrot.

3 Add all the ingredients into a blender.

4 Blitz well until smooth.

CHEF'S NOTE
A smoothie that tastes like cake has to be a fantastic way to kick start your morning. This smoothie is bursting with antioxidants and healthy fats.

BAKED BANANA PORRIDGE

Ingredients

- 2 small bananas, halved lengthways
- 100g jumbo porridge oats
- ¼ tsp cinnamon
- 150ml milk of your choice, plus extra to serve
- 4 roughly chopped walnuts

Method

1 Preheat the oven to 190C/375F/gas 5.

2 Mash up one banana half, then mix it with the oats, cinnamon, milk, 300ml water and a pinch of salt, and pour into a baking dish.

3 Top with the remaining banana halves and scatter over the walnuts.

4 Bake for 20-25 mins until the oats are creamy and have absorbed most of the liquid.

CHEF'S NOTE

This may seem a touch involved for a weekday morning, but the prep is minimal and can be done the night before, leaving you enough time to jump in the shower while it bakes.

MEXICAN BREAKFAST

Ingredients

- 140g/4½oz quartered cherry tomatoes
- 1 finely chopped red onion
- Juice of ½ a lime
- 2 tbsp olive oil
- 1 crushed garlic cloves
- 1 tsp ground cumin
- 1 tsp chipotle paste
- 1 x 400g/14oz tin of black beans, drained
- Small chopped bunch of coriander
- 2 slices wholemeal bread
- 1 finely sliced avocado

Method

1 Mix the tomatoes, ¼ onion, lime juice and 1 tbsp oil and set aside. Fry the remaining onion in 1 tbsp oil until it starts to soften. Add the garlic, fry for 1 min, then add the cumin and chipotle paste and stir to combine.

2 Tip in the beans and a splash of water, stir and cook gently until heated through. Stir in most of the tomato mixture, cook for 1 min. Season well, and add most of the coriander.

3 Toast the bread and drizzle with the remaining 1 tbsp oil. Place a slice on a plate and pile some beans on top. Arrange some slices of avocado on top, then sprinkle with the remaining tomato mixture and coriander leaves to serve.

CHEF'S NOTE

Arriba! This Mexican feast is bursting with fresh, vibrant flavours that will kick start your palate and metabolism for the day, leaving you full and well-nourished.

NUT BUTTER CRÊPES

Ingredients

- 75g/3oz gluten-free brown bread flour
- 1 tsp ground cinnamon
- 1 medium egg
- 225ml/8 fl oz semi-skimmed milk
- 1 tsp rapeseed oil
- 2 tbsp nut butter of your choice
- 1 sliced banana
- A handful of berries of your choice

Method

1 Tip the flour into a large mixing bowl with the cinnamon. Add the egg and milk, and whisk vigorously until you have a smooth pouring consistency.

2 Place a non-stick frying pan over a medium heat and add a little of the oil. When it begins to heat, wipe most of it away with kitchen paper.

3 Once the pan is hot, pour a small amount of the batter into the centre of the pan and swirl it to the sides in a thin layer. Leave to cook, untouched, for about 2 mins. When it is brown underneath, turn over and cook for 1 min more.

4 Transfer to a warm plate and cover with foil to keep warm. Repeat with the remaining batter.

5 Divide the warm pancakes between 2 plates and serve with the nut butter, banana and berries of your choosing.

CHEF'S NOTE
Nut butters are a delicious way to get protein and healthy fats into your diet. Different varieties taste different and go well with different things so why not branch out from peanut butter and try hazelnut or cashew?

LUNCH
RECIPES

AVOCADO CHICKEN SALAD

Ingredients

- 1 cooked chicken breast shredded or chopped
- 1 ripe avocado pitted and diced
- 125g/4oz tinned sweetcorn
- 1 small chopped red or green pepper

- 1 tbsp chopped coriander
- 1 tbsp lime juice
- 1 tbsp olive oil

Method

1 In a large bowl, add the shredded chicken, avocado, onion, pepper, sweetcorn and coriander.

2 Squeeze over the lime juice, olive oil.

3 Season with salt and pepper. Toss gently until all the ingredients are combined and serve.

CHEF'S NOTE

Avocados are full of healthy fats that will help keep you satisfied. This salad works well with leftover roast chicken or with added black beans, tomato (nightshades permitting) and even chopped bacon.

VEGETABLE BUDDHA BOWL

Ingredients

- 125g/4oz quartered button mushrooms
- 175g/6oz cooked quinoa or wholegrain rice
- 125g/4oz red peppers
- 125g/4oz yellow peppers
- 125g/4oz cooked or pickled red cabbage
- 125g/4oz sun dried tomatoes
- 125g/4oz grilled Brussels sprouts
- ½ sweet potato
- 60ml/2fl oz olive oil

Method

1 Preheat your oven to 190C/gas 5/375F

2 Using large baking pan, drizzle olive oil, salt and pepper over the mushrooms, peppers and Brussels sprouts.

3 Pierce the sweet potato and bake in the oven with the vegetables for 30 mins or until soft.

4 Build your bowl by adding the mushrooms, peppers, cabbage, sun dried tomatoes, quinoa or rice and Brussels sprouts with the baked sweet potato perched on top.

CHEF'S NOTE

This bowl is fully of fresh flavours, low GI, vegan and infinitely adaptable. Feel free to swap the veg and grains for your personal favourites and squeeze with lemon for some extra tang!

31

SPICED SWEET POTATO SOUP

Ingredients

- 1 tsp olive oil
- A pinch of cumin seeds
- A pinch of coriander seeds
- A pinch of turmeric
- A pinch of chilli flakes
- A pinch of ground cinnamon
- A pinch of paprika
- ½ red onion, finely chopped
- ½ sweet potato, peeled and chopped
- 200ml/7fl oz vegetable stock

Method

1 Heat the oil in a saucepan over a medium heat and add all of the spices.

2 Add the onion and sweet potato and cook for around 3 minutes ,then add the vegetable stock.

3 Turn down the heat and cook for a further 8-10 minutes, or until the potato is soft.

4 Leave the soup chunky, or blitz in a blender until smooth, and serve in a large bowl.

CHEF'S NOTE
Soup is a perfect lunch or late supper. Increase quantities and freeze in portions. A flask filled with boiling water in the morning before being discarded and replaced with warm soup will stay warm until lunchtime.

THAI CHICKEN SALAD

Ingredients

- 1 head Chinese leaf or ½ iceberg lettuce, shredded
- 2 cooked chicken breasts or 200g leftover cooked chicken, shredded
- 1 mango, peeled, stoned and thinly sliced
- Leaves from a bunch of mint
- 6 spring onions, sliced diagonally
- 3 tbsp salted peanuts, roughly chopped

For the dressing:
- Juice of 4 limes
- 4 tbsp sesame oil
- A splash of fish sauce
- 2 large red chillies, deseeded and finely chopped

Method

1 First make the dressing by mixing together all the ingredients along with 2 tsp sugar.

2 Then in a large bowl, mix all the salad ingredients except the nuts.

3 Toss with the dressing and season with black pepper. Scatter the nuts on top to serve.

CHEF'S NOTE
The balance of sweet, spicy, hot and sour flavours and soft, crisp and crunchy textures make this an addictive salad. Make sure your fish sauce is gluten free if you are intolerant.

VIETNAMESE SEAFOOD NOODLES

Ingredients

- 400g/14oz pack cooked seafood mix
- 300g/11oz pack cooked thin brown rice noodles
- 300g/11oz cooked beansprouts
- 3 carrots, thinly sliced
- 1 bunch spring onions, sliced lengthways
- A bunch mint and coriander, leaves chopped

For the dressing:
- 5 tbsp rice wine vinegar
- 1 tsp caster sugar
- 1 red chilli, chopped
- 1 stick lemongrass, sliced
- 1 soy sauce

Method

1 To make the salad put all of the vegetables and seafood in a large bowl and mix everything together, so that the seafood and noodles are combined.

2 Then make the dressing by mixing all of the ingredients and toss this through the salad before serving.

CHEF'S NOTE
High in iodine and zinc from the seafood and salty soy, this salad makes a hearty, yet fresh meal. Brown rice noodles keep this low GI, it's great for sharing and travels well in a lunchbox for picnicking or a desk-bound lunch.

SALMON, LEMON AND BROWN RICE SALAD

Ingredients

- 200g/7oz brown basmati rice
- 200g/7oz frozen soya beans, defrosted
- 2 salmon fillets
- 1 cucumber, diced
- 1 small bunch spring onion, sliced

- 1 small bunch coriander, roughly chopped
- Zest and juice 1 lime
- 1 red chilli, diced (deseeded if you like it mild)
- 4 tsp light soy sauce

Method

1 Cook the rice following the pack instructions and 3 mins before it's done, add the soya beans. Drain and cool under cold running water.

2 Meanwhile, put the salmon on a plate, then microwave on high for 3 mins, or until cooked through. Allow to cool slightly, remove the skin with a fork, then flake.

3 Gently fold the cucumber, spring onions, coriander and salmon into the rice and beans. In a separate bowl, mix the lime zest and juice, chilli and soy sauce then pour over the rice before serving.

CHEF'S NOTE
This dish is packed full of healthy fats, protein and omega 3 from the salmon. The brown rice and fish will help stabilise your blood sugar levels, keeping you full for longer.

ROASTED CHICKPEA WRAP

Ingredients

- 1 400g/14oz can chickpeas
- 1 tsp olive oil
- 1 tsp ground cumin
- 1 tsp smoked paprika
- 1 stoned peeled and chopped avocado
- Juice 1 lime

- Small bunch of chopped coriander
- 4 soft corn or wholemeal tortillas
- ½ small iceberg lettuce, shredded
- 75g/3oz natural yogurt
- 250g/9oz jar roasted red peppers, chopped

Method

1 Heat your oven to 220C/425F/Gas 7.

2 Drain the chickpeas and put in a large bowl. Add the olive oil, cumin and paprika. Stir the chickpeas well to coat, then spread them onto a large baking tray and roast for 20-25 mins, or until starting to go crisp – give the tray a shake halfway through cooking to ensure they roast evenly. Remove from the oven and season to taste.

3 Toss the chopped avocados with the lime juice and chopped coriander, then set aside until serving. Warm the tortillas following pack instructions, then pile in the avocado, lettuce, yogurt, peppers and toasted chickpeas at the table.

CHEF'S NOTE

This tasty lunchtime treat is full of protein and healthy fats and is great for vegetarians, if you're vegan, swap the natural yogurt for coconut cream or pureed silken tofu.

BEEF AND BARLEY BROTH

Ingredients

- 2 tsp olive oil
- 500g/1lb 2oz diced stewing steak
- 1 tbsp Marmite or vegemite
- 1 splash of Worcestershire sauce
- 1 red onion
- 2 carrots

- 3 sticks of celery
- 1 fresh bay leaf
- 1 sprig of fresh rosemary
- 1 tbsp plain flour
- 2l/3pts beef stock
- 150g/5oz pearl barley

Method

1 Warm the olive oil in a large pan over a medium heat. Add the steak and cook until the meat is lightly browned all over.

2 Stir in the Marmite and Worcestershire sauce, turn the heat up to high and keep stirring until all the liquid has evaporated.

3 Meanwhile, peel and chop the onion, carrots and celery.

4 Add the chopped veg to the pan with the bay leaf and rosemary sprig and cook over a low heat with the lid on, until softened.

5 Stir in the flour and, after 1 minute, pour in the stock. Season well with sea salt and black pepper.

6 Bring to the boil, then reduce to a simmer, add the pearl barley and cook gently for 1 hour, then remove from the heat and discard the rosemary sprig and bay leaf.

CHEF'S NOTE

This soup takes a while to prepare so it's good to make a big batch at the weekend. It's hearty broth that's perfect for the winter months. Serve with wholemeal bread for a comforting supper.

TUNA AND BEAN SALAD

Ingredients

- 1 carrot, peeled and coarsely grated
- 1 red pepper, deseeded and sliced
- 100g/3½oz sugar snap peas, finely sliced
- 400g/14oz tinned cannellini or butter beans

- 125g/4oz salad leaves
- 3 tbsp of your favourite salad dressing, bought or homemade
- 200g/7oz tinned tuna in brine, drained

Method

1 Mix the carrot, pepper, sugar snap peas and beans together in a large bowl.

2 Gently toss in the salad leaves and half of the dressing, then flake the tuna over.

3 Drizzle with a little more dressing when you serve.

CHEF'S NOTE

Fresh, vibrant and packed with flavour. The tuna is a good source of selenium and the beans contain high levels of zinc, both shown to help maintain a healthy thyroid.

BAKED SWEET POTATO

Ingredients

- 1 medium sweet potato
- 1 tsp olive oil
- Zest and juice of ½ lemon
- 40g/1½oz natural yoghurt
- A pinch of turmeric
- A pinch of ground cumin

- 1 small carrot
- 2-3 radishes
- ½ raw beetroots
- ¼ red onion
- ¼ apple

Method

1 Preheat the oven to 180°C/350°F/Gas 4.

2 Scrub the potato, pat dry, then rub with a little olive oil, a pinch of sea salt and black pepper. Roast on a baking tray for about 40 minutes, or until cooked through.

3 Finely grate half the lemon zest into a small bowl and mix in the yoghurt, turmeric and cumin. Leave at room temperature until needed.

4 Scrub the carrots, radishes and beetroot, peel the onion and core the apple. Push through the grating blade of your food processor, or coarsely grate by hand, then tip into a bowl.

5 Cut a cross in the top of your cooked potato and gently break it open with a fork, mashing a little of the inside as you go.

6 Spoon over a good dollop of the spiced yoghurt, followed by the grated salad.

CHEF'S NOTE

Sweet potatoes are a great lower-GI alternative to regular potatoes. The salad and spiced yoghurt topping works well with the sweet flesh, but can be swapped for your own favourite.

39

CHICKEN SOUP

Ingredients

- 55g/2oz butter
- 2 onions, sliced
- 2 sticks celery, finely chopped
- 2 carrots, finely diced
- 25g/2oz plain flour

- 1.2l/2pts chicken stock
- 450g/1lb cooked chicken, shredded
- 1 tbsp chopped fresh parsley

Method

1 Melt the butter in a large saucepan over a medium heat and gently fry the onions, celery and carrots until they start to soften.

2 Stir in the flour and cook for 2 minutes. Add the chicken stock and bring the mixture to the boil, stirring as you do so. Season with salt and pepper, then reduce the heat and simmer for 10 minutes, until the vegetables are tender.

3 Add the cooked chicken until heated through. Adjust the seasoning, stir in the parsley and serve.

CHEF'S NOTE

In Jewish culture, chicken soup is seen as a panacea - curing all ills both physical and emotional. This easy to make version will nurture your body and soul.

PASTA SALAD GREEK-STYLE

Ingredients

- 75g/3oz whole wheat pasta, such as penne or conchiglie
- ½ unwaxed lemon, finely grated zest and juice
- ¼ red onion, finely chopped
- ½ tbsp olive oil, ideally extra virgin

- ¼ cucumber, peeled and cubed
- 100g/3½oz cherry tomatoes, quartered
- 1 tbsp fresh basil, roughly chopped
- 75g/3oz feta, crumbled (optional)
- Handful pitted black olives (optional)
- Sea salt and freshly ground black pepper

Method

1 Cook the pasta in a saucepan of boiling, salted water as per the packet instructions.

2 Whisk together the lemon zest and juice, red onion, oil and a generous amount of pepper.

3 Drain the pasta in a colander and run it under a cold tap until cooled.

4 Stir the dressing, cucumber, tomatoes, basil, feta and olives, if using, into the pasta and serve.

CHEF'S NOTE

This recipe will not be suitable if you're following a paleo diet, but using whole wheat pasta keeps this recipe low GI and healthy.

TUNA LETTUCE WRAPS

Ingredients

- 2 drops rapeseed oil
- 2 x 140g/4½oz tuna fillets
- 1 ripe avocado
- ½ tsp English mustard powder

- 1 tsp cider vinegar
- 1 tbsp capers
- 8 romaine lettuce leaves
- 16 halved cherry tomatoes

Method

1 Brush the tuna with a little oil. Heat a non-stick pan, add the tuna and cook for 1 min each side, or a min or so longer for a thicker fillet. Transfer to a plate to rest.

2 Halve and stone the avocado and scoop the flesh into a small bowl. Add the mustard powder and vinegar, then mash well so that the mixture is smooth like mayonnaise. Stir in the capers. Spoon into two small dishes and put on serving plates with the lettuce leaves, and tomatoes.

3 Slice the tuna (it should be slightly pink inside) and arrange on the plates. Spoon some 'mayo' on the lettuce leaves and top with tuna and cherry tomatoes and a few extra capers. To eat, roll up into little wraps.

CHEF'S NOTE

If you're following a paleo or autoimmune paleo diet (AIP) then replacing slices of bread with lettuce is a good way of enjoying your usual fillings. This also works well as a wrap replacement for fajitas.

TORTILLA

Ingredients

- 300g/11oz waxy potatoes
- 1 onion, sliced
- Olive oil
- 5 large free-range eggs

Method

1 Peel the potatoes and cut into thin slices.

2 Peel and finely slice the onion. Drizzle 2 tbsp of oil into a small frying pan over a medium heat, then add the onion and potatoes.

3 Turn the heat down to low and cook for 25 to 30 mins, or until the onions are turning golden and the potato slices are cooked through. Try not to stir it too much or the potatoes will break up.

4 Crack the eggs into a mixing bowl, season and mix together with a fork.

5 Add the eggs to the frying pan and place it over a low heat. Cook for around 20 mins, or until there's almost no runny egg on top.

6 Use a fish slice to slightly lift and loosen the sides of the tortilla. Carefully flip the pan over a dinner plate and tip out the tortilla, then slide it back into the pan and cook for another 5 minutes, or until golden and cooked through.

CHEF'S NOTE

A tortilla, or Spanish omelette, has the advantage of being able to be eaten hot or cold. Why not have it warm for dinner and then have the leftovers cold the next day?

CHICKEN FATTOUSH

Ingredients

- Juice of 1 lemon
- 1 tbsp olive oil
- ½ Cos lettuce, chopped
- 1 large tomato, chopped into chunks
- ½ small pack flat-leaf parsley, chopped
- ½ cucumber, chopped into chunks
- 125g/4oz cooked chicken
- 1 sliced spring onion
- 1 wholemeal pitta bread
- 1-2 tsp ground sumac

Method

1 Pour the lemon juice into a large bowl and whisk while slowly adding the oil. When all the oil has been added, and the mixture starts to thicken, season.

2 Add the lettuce, tomatoes, parsley, cucumber, chicken pieces and spring onions, and stir well to coat the salad in the dressing.

3 Put the pitta bread in the toaster until crisp and golden, then chop into chunks. Scatter the toasted pitta pieces over the salad and sprinkle over the sumac. Serve straight away.

CHEF'S NOTE

Using bread in a salad may seem unusual but like the Italian Panzanella, this salad is bulked out by using it. The wholemeal pita is low GI and will keep you full with stabilized blood sugar levels.

UDON NOODLE SOUP

Ingredients

- 1 vegetable stock cube
- 60ml/1fl oz teriyaki sauce
- 1 tbsp vegetable oil
- 140g/4½oz chestnut mushroom, sliced
- ½ bunch spring onions, thinly sliced
- 140g/4½oz wholemeal udon noodles
- 200g/7oz spinach

Method

1 In a large pan, dissolve the stock cube in 1 litre of water and stir in the teriyaki sauce.

2 While the soup base comes to the boil, heat the oil in a frying pan and cook the mushrooms over a high heat for 2-3 mins, until they turn golden. Add the spring onions and cook for 1 min more, then set aside.

3 Once the soup base has come to the boil, add the noodles and cook for 4 mins. Add the spinach and cook for 1 min more until they are just wilted. Stir in the mushrooms, spring onions and some seasoning. Serve.

CHEF'S NOTE
Udon noodles are thicker than usual egg noodles, and will keep you feeling fuller for longer. For an extra protein boost consider adding some cooked chicken, prawns or tofu.

SALMON OPEN SANDWICH

Ingredients

- 2 slices of wholemeal or granary bread
- 1 lemon, halved
- 1 small avocado
- A few dill sprigs, plus extra to serve
- 1 small red onion, ½ sliced, the rest finely chopped
- 2 skinless, boneless wild salmon fillets

Method

1 Bring a small pan of water to the boil and add a good squeeze of lemon, a few dill sprigs and the sliced onion. Add the salmon and leave to poach for 8-10 mins or until it flakes easily. Lift from the pan and flake into small pieces.

2 Scoop the avocado into a bowl and roughly mash with a generous squeeze of lemon.

3 Top the bread with the avocado, scatter over half the chopped onion, then top with salmon, more onions and some snipped dill. Squeeze over some lemon to serve.

CHEF'S NOTE

Sandwiches are an easy go-to for lunch, but can be carb-heavy, making us feel sluggish. Having an open sandwich with only one slice of bread helps lighten the meal.

DINNER
RECIPES

BAKED TROUT

Ingredients

- 2 large carrots, cut into batons
- 3 celery sticks, cut into batons
- 1 tbsp olive oil
- 6 tbsp white wine vinegar
- Two 175g/6oz trout fillets
- Basil leaves
- Juice 1 lemon

Method

1 Heat oven to 190C/375F/gas 5. Put the carrots and celery in a pan with the oil, vinegar, salt and pepper. Bring to the boil, tightly cover, then cook for 10 mins, until the vegetables are tender. Drain and put to one side.

2 Cut two large sheets of baking parchment, about 35cm square. Divide the vegetables between them and top each with a trout fillet. Scatter a few basil leaves and a little lemon juice over each, then season the fish with a little salt and pepper. Fold the paper in half and double fold all round to seal in the trout, a bit like a pasty.

3 Put the parcels on two baking sheets and bake for 15-20 mins (depending on the thickness of the fish). Serve in their paper with some steamed new potatoes.

CHEF'S NOTE
This dish is naturally gluten free and suitable for am AIP adapted diet (if served without potatoes) and is delicious and sophisticated enough to serve at a dinner party.

BEAN BURGERS

Ingredients

- 50g/2oz pine nuts
- 425g/15oz tinned borlotti beans, drained and rinsed
- 1 small red onion, finely chopped
- 2 tbsp sundried tomato paste
- 75g/3oz ground almonds
- 1 tbsp fresh thyme leaves
- 1 beaten egg
- Sunflower oil, for frying

To serve:
- Tzatziki, mayonnaise or natural yoghurt
- Iceberg lettuce leaves

Method

1 Place a frying pan over a medium heat and lightly toast the pine nuts for 2-3 mins or until golden. Remove from pan and set to one side.

2 Put the borlotti beans into a large bowl and mash well with a potato masher or fork. Add the pine nuts, onion, tomato paste, half of the ground almonds, the thyme and egg. Season to taste, then gently mix together until the ingredients are thoroughly combined.

3 With slightly wet hands, shape the mixture into 4 burgers. Coat the outside of each burger with the remaining almonds. Cover and chill in the fridge for at least 30 mins.

4 To cook the burgers: heat a thin layer of sunflower oil in a large frying pan and fry for 3-4 mins each side, until golden. Drain on kitchen paper, then serve wrapped in iceberg lettuce leaves and spoon over the sauce of your choice.

CHEF'S NOTE

Burgers can be a difficult food to eat if you have thyroid issues. This version is just as tasty, but with no breadcrumb binder and no bun. The beans make this high in zinc.

KALE AND SALMON KEDGEREE

Ingredients

- 150g/5oz brown rice
- 1 medium salmon fillet
- 2 eggs
- 1 tbsp vegetable oil
- 50g/2oz curly kale, stalks removed, roughly chopped

- 1 onion, finely chopped
- 1 garlic clove, crushed
- 1 tbsp curry powder
- 1 tsp turmeric
- Zest and juice ½ lemon

Method

1 Cook the rice following pack instructions. Meanwhile, season the salmon and steam over a pan of simmering water for 8 mins, or until just cooked. Keep the pan of water on the heat, add the eggs and boil for 6 mins, then run under cold water.

2 Heat the oil in a large frying pan or wok, add the onion and cook for 5 mins. Throw in the kale and cook, stirring, for 5 mins. Add the garlic, curry powder, turmeric and rice, then season and stir until heated through.

3 Peel and quarter the eggs. Flake the salmon and gently fold through the rice, then divide between plates and top with the eggs. Sprinkle over the lemon zest and squeeze over a little juice before serving.

CHEF'S NOTE

Traditionally an Anglo-Indian breakfast dish, this combination of spiced rice and fish make a delicious dinner. The brown rice and kale make this a healthy, low GI dish.

LEMON COD WITH BEAN MASH

Ingredients

- 2 small bunches cherry tomatoes, on the vine
- 1 tbsp olive oil
- 2 skinless cod, or other white fish, fillets
- Zest and juice 1 lemon
- 250g/9oz pack frozen soya beans
- 1 garlic clove
- 1 small bunch of basil, leaves and stalks separated
- 100ml/3½fl oz chicken or vegetable stock

Method

1 Heat your oven to 200C/fan 400F/gas 6. Put the tomatoes onto a baking tray, rub with a little oil and some seasoning, then roast for 5 mins until the skins are starting to split. Add the fish to the tray, top with most of the lemon zest and some more seasoning, then drizzle with a little more oil. Roast for 8-10 mins until the fish flakes easily.

2 Meanwhile, cook the beans in a pan of boiling water for 3 mins, until just tender. Drain, then tip into a food processor with the rest of the oil, garlic, basil stalks, lemon juice and stock, then pulse to a thick, slightly rough purée. Season to taste.

3 Divide the tomatoes and mash between two plates, top with the cod, then scatter with basil leaves and the remaining lemon zest to serve.

CHEF'S NOTE

Mashing or blending vegetables in this way makes a great alternative to having potatoes. Try experimenting with different varieties, such as peas or broccoli.

MOROCCAN MEATBALLS

Ingredients

- 1 small onion, finely chopped
- 2 tbsp olive oil
- 25g/1oz ground almonds
- 250g/9oz pack lean lamb mince
- ½ tsp ground cinnamon
- 3 eggs
- 2 garlic cloves, sliced

- 1 courgette, thickly sliced
- 400g/14oz tinned chopped tomatoes
- 1 tsp honey
- 1 tsp ras el hanout spice mix
- A small bunch of coriander, mostly chopped
- 400g/14oz tinned chickpeas, rinsed & drained

Method

1 Fry the onion in 1 tbsp oil until soft, then allow to cool. Mix with the almonds, mince, cinnamon, 1 egg, ½ tsp salt and lots of pepper. Then, with wet hands, shape into about 12 meatballs.

2 Fry in the remaining oil in a shallow pan for about 8 mins, moving them round until evenly browned. Lift out and set aside.

3 Add the garlic to the oil left in the pan and fry until softened. Add the courgette, fry for 1-2 mins, then tip in the tomatoes, honey, ras el hanout, three-quarters of the coriander, seasoning and a couple of tbsp water. Stir and cook until soft and pulpy.

4 Stir in the chickpeas and add the meatballs. Make 2 hollows in the sauce, then break in the remaining eggs. Cover and cook for 4-8 mins over a low heat until the eggs are set. Scatter with coriander and serve straight from the pan.

CHEF'S NOTE

This one pot meal has something in common with the middle eastern egg recipe in the breakfast section, but the meatballs and Moroccan spices make it taste quite different.

PESTO FISH GRATIN

Ingredients

- 2 chunky white fish fillets
- 2 slices prosciutto
- 100g/3½oz crème fraîche
- 1 ½ tbsp pesto
- 25g/1oz grated Parmesan
- 1 tbsp pine nuts

Method

1 Heat oven to 200C/400F/fan/gas 6. Season the fish all over, then wrap each fillet in a slice of prosciutto.

2 Put into a large baking dish. Dot the crème fraîche between the fillets and over the exposed ends of the fish. Dot the pesto around the fish, too. Scatter with the cheese.

3 Bake the fish for 15-20 mins, adding the pine nuts halfway through, until the crème fraîche has made a sauce around the fish, and the cheese and ham are turning golden.

CHEF'S NOTE

Full of healthy fats, this delicious dish goes well when served with streamed green vegetables or boiled peas - perfect for soaking up the tasty sauce.

SPANISH FISH STEW

Ingredients

- Handful flat-leaf parsley leaves, chopped
- 1 garlic clove, finely chopped
- Zest and juice 1 lemon
- 2 tbsp olive oil
- 1 small onion, finely sliced
- 250g/9oz floury potatoes, cut into small chunks
- 1 tsp paprika
- Pinch cayenne pepper
- 400g/14fl oz tinned of chopped tomatoes
- 1 fish stock cube
- 100g/3½oz raw peeled king prawns
- 200g/7oz tinned chickpeas, rinsed and drained
- 250g/9oz skinless fish fillets, cut into very large chunks

Method

1 In a small bowl, mix the parsley with ½ the garlic and lemon zest, then set aside. Heat 2 tbsp oil in a large sauté pan. Throw in the onion and potatoes, cover the pan, then sweat everything for about 5 mins until the onion has softened. Add the remaining oil, garlic and spices, then cook for 2 mins more.

2 Pour over the lemon juice and sizzle for a moment. Add the tomatoes and crumble in the stock. Season with a little salt, then cover the pan. Simmer everything for 15-20 mins, until the potatoes are just cooked.

3 Stir through the prawns and chickpeas, then nestle the fish chunks into the top of the stew. Reduce the heat and re-cover the pan, then cook for about 8 mins, stirring very gently once or twice.

4 When the fish is just cooked through, remove from the heat, scatter with the parsley mix and serve with some crusty bread, if you can tolerate it.

CHEF'S NOTE
This recipe is easy to scale up, or can be adapted to use chicken instead of fish. If you avoid gluten then check your stock cube to ensure they're suitable.

MOZZARELLA CHICKEN WITH BUTTER BEAN MASH

Ingredients

- 2 chicken breasts
- Olive oil
- 1 small onion, thinly sliced
- 1 crushed garlic clove
- 400g/14oz tinned chopped tomatoes
- 2 tbsp tomato purée

- 1 tsp dried oregano
- 75g/3oz pitted green or black olives
- 125g/4oz reduced fat mozzarella, sliced and drained
- For the mash:
- 1 small onion, finely chopped
- 1 garlic clove, crushed

- 400g/14oz tinned butter beans, drained
- A good squeeze of lemon juice

Method

1 Season the chicken breasts with salt and pepper. Add a little oil to a frying pan and place over a high heat. Cook the chicken on each side for 3 minutes, or until lightly browned. Transfer to a plate.

2 Reduce the heat to low, add a little more oil into the pan and cook the onion for 4-5 minutes, stirring until softened and lightly browned. Add the garlic and cook for a few seconds.

3 Pour in the tomatoes. Stir in the tomato purée, oregano, olives and 150ml/5fl oz cold water. Bring to the boil and cook for 5 minutes, stirring regularly. Reduce the heat to a gentle simmer and add the chicken. Cook for 10 minutes, until the chicken is tender and cooked through.

4 Preheat the grill. Top the chicken and sauce with the sliced mozzarella. Sprinkle with black pepper and cook for 2 mins or until the cheese melts.

5 For the butter bean mash, add a little oil to a saucepan and place over a medium heat. Add the onion and cook for 3 minutes. Add the garlic and cook for a further minute.

6 Put the beans in a food processor with 100ml/3½fl oz water, and a good pinch of salt and pepper. Add the cooked onion and garlic, and blend to a thick purée. Spoon back in to the saucepan and heat, stirring constantly until hot. Add a good squeeze of lemon and season to taste.

7 Divide the butterbean mash between 2 plates and add the chicken and sauce. Serve with freshly cooked vegetables or salad.

LAMB TAGINE

Ingredients

- 600g/1lb 5oz lean lamb leg steaks, cut into bite-size cubes
- 1–2 level tbsp harissa paste
- 400g/14oz tinned chopped tomatoes with herbs
- 2 x 400g/14oz tinned chickpeas, drained
- 12 dried apricots (optional)
- Small bunch (about 30g/1oz) fresh coriander, roughly chopped

Method

1 Preheat the oven to 170C/325F/Gas 3

2 Put the lamb in a medium, ovenproof casserole dish or tagine and coat evenly with the harissa paste.

3 Pour in the tomatoes and 300ml/10floz of water. Bring to the boil over a medium heat and stir well.

4 Cover tightly with kitchen foil if using a casserole dish, or place the lid on a tagine and bake for 1 hour.

5 Stir in the chickpeas and apricots, if using, and bake for 30–45 minutes, or until the lamb is tender.

6 Stir in the coriander and serve.

CHEF'S NOTE

This dish is gluten free, contains high levels of protein and is low on the glycemic index. Lamb makes a lovely alternative to everyday chicken when dining at the weekend.

CHICKEN CURRY

Ingredients

- Cooking oil spray
- 2 onions, finely chopped
- 6-8 chicken thighs, boned, skinned and trimmed.
- 2 garlic cloves, crushed
- 20g/¾oz ginger, finely grated
- 2 tsp garam masala

- ½ tsp hot chilli powder
- 400g/14oz tinned chopped tomatoes
- 600ml/1 pint chicken stock, 100g/3½oz dried red split lentils, rinsed and drained
- 2 bay leaves

- 200g/7oz wholegrain long grain rice
- To serve:
- 150g/5½oz fat-free natural yoghurt
- 1 tbsp roughly chopped fresh coriander leaves

Method

1 Spray a wide-based saucepan or sauté pan with oil and place over a medium heat. Cook the onions for 5 minutes, stirring regularly, until softened and very lightly browned.

2 Cut the chicken thighs in half and add to the pan. Cook for 2 minutes, turning occasionally. Stir in the garlic, ginger, garam masala and chilli powder and cook for a few seconds, stirring constantly.

3 Tip the tomatoes into the pan and add the chicken stock, lentils and bay leaves. Bring to the boil, then cover loosely with a lid and simmer gently for 35 minutes, or until the chicken is tender and the lentils have completely broken down, stirring occasionally. Remove the lid for the last 10 minutes of cooking time, stirring regularly so the lentils don't stick.

4 About 25 minutes before the curry is ready, cook the rice in plenty of boiling water until tender, then drain well.

5 Season the curry to taste. Serve with the rice, topped with yoghurt and sprinkled with coriander.

CHEF'S NOTE

Takeaways can be difficult when you're regulating your diet, as it's hard to always know what is in it. Make your own for a tastier and healthier option.

TROUT WRAPPED IN BACON

Ingredients

- 2 trout fillets
- 2 strips thick cut bacon
- Juice of 1 lemon

- 2 sprigs thyme
- Green salad to serve

Method

1 Season the fish and sprinkle with thyme leaves, squeeze the lemon over the fillets.

2 Wrap each fish in the bacon and fry in a hot pan for around 3 mins a side, or until the bacon is crispy.

3 Serve immediately with a green salad garnish.

CHEF'S NOTE
Trout is an oily fish, full of omega 3. This tasty and simple dish is high in selenium, quick and easy, so perfect for a speedy midweek supper.

CHICKPEA, SPINACH AND EGG CURRY

Ingredients

- 2 large free-range eggs
- 1 tbsp light olive oil
- 2 tsp cumin seeds
- 1 tsp black mustard seeds
- 2 tbsp medium curry powder, plus extra for sprinkling

- 1 tsp garlic granules
- 1 tsp ground ginger
- 400g/14oz tinned chopped tomatoes
- 400g/14oz tinned chickpeas, drained and rinsed

- 1 tbsp lemon juice
- 100ml/3½fl oz boiling water
- 175g/6oz baby leaf spinach
- salt and freshly ground black pepper
- 2 tbsp chopped fresh coriander to garnish

Method

1 Bring a small saucepan of water to the boil and cook the eggs for 6–8 minutes, or until done to your liking. When cool enough to handle remove the shells, halve and set aside.

2 Meanwhile, heat the oil in a wide frying pan over a low heat. Add the cumin, black mustard seeds, curry powder, garlic granules and ground ginger and stir-fry for 1 minute.

3 Add the tomatoes, chickpeas, lemon juice and boiling water, then season with salt and pepper. Cook over a high heat for 6–8 minutes, or until reduced and thickened, stirring often. Add the spinach and cook until wilted.

4 Divide the curry between two shallow bowls, top each with two egg halves and sprinkle over some curry powder. Scatter with coriander and serve immediately.

CHEF'S NOTE

This vegetarian, gluten free dish may have a long list of ingredients but you may have most in your spice rack. It takes only 20 mins to cook, so perfect for a midweek meal.

SALMON WITH PUY LENTILS

Ingredients

- 200g/7oz Puy lentils
- 1 bay leaf
- 200g/7oz fine green beans, chopped
- 25g/1oz flat leaf parsley, chopped
- 2 tbsp Dijon mustard
- 2 tbsp capers, rinsed and chopped

- 2 tbsp olive oil
- 2 lemons, finely sliced
- 500g/1lb 2oz salmon fillets
- 1 fennel bulb, finely sliced
- Dill sprigs, to garnish
- Salt and freshly ground black pepper

Method

1 Put the lentils in a saucepan with the bay leaf and enough cold water to cover. Bring to the boil, reduce to a simmer and cook for 30 minutes, or until tender. Season to taste with salt and freshly ground black pepper. Add the beans and simmer for a further minute.

2 Drain the lentils and discard the bay leaf. Stir in the parsley, mustard, capers and oil.

3 Preheat the grill to a hot setting.

4 Arrange the lemon slices on a foil-lined grill pan and place the salmon and fennel slices on top. Season the salmon and fennel with salt and freshly ground black pepper.

5 Cook under the grill for about 10 minutes, or until the salmon is cooked through.

6 Place the salmon on top of the lentils and fennel slices, garnish with dill sprigs and serve.

CHEF'S NOTE
Lentils are a nutritionally dense food, rich in zinc. They're also relatively cheap, so why not try introducing them in your diet as a side dish or as the 'star of the show' in a dal or lentil soup.

RED MULLET WITH ROAST TOMATOES

Ingredients

- 375g/13oz mixed red and yellow cherry tomatoes
- 350g/12oz fine green beans, trimmed
- 2 garlic cloves, finely chopped
- 2 tbsp lemon juice
- Low-calorie cooking spray

- Salt and freshly ground black pepper
- 8 red mullet fillets, approximately 100g/3½oz each
- 1 lemon, finely grated rind only
- 2 tsp baby capers, drained
- 2 spring onions, finely sliced

Method

1 Preheat the oven to 200C/400F/Gas 6.

2 Put the tomatoes in an ovenproof dish with the beans, garlic and lemon juice then spray with the oil. Season with salt and freshly ground black pepper and mix well. Bake for 10 minutes, or until the tomatoes and beans are tender.

3 Meanwhile, tear off 4 large sheets of foil and line with non-stick baking paper. Place 2 fish fillets on each piece of baking paper, then scatter over the lemon zest, capers and spring onions. Season with salt and freshly ground black pepper. Fold over the paper-lined foil and scrunch the edges together to seal. Place the parcels on a large baking tray.

4 Place the fish parcels next to the vegetables in the oven and bake for a further 8-10 minutes, or until the flesh flakes easily when pressed in the centre with a knife.

5 Spoon the vegetables on to four serving plates, top each with two fish fillets and serve.

CHEF'S NOTE
Although not suitable for anyone with a sensitivity to nightshade vegetables, this meal is paleo friendly, gluten free and deliciously tasty!

AUBERGINE PARMIGIANA

Ingredients

- 6 large beefsteak tomatoes - tops sliced off a quarter of the way down the tomato and reserved, seeds and pulp scooped out and reserved
- 9 tbsp extra virgin olive oil, plus extra for drizzling
- 1 small onion, peeled & chopped

- 2 handfuls fresh basil leaves
- 2-3 tbsp plain flour
- 400g/14oz small aubergines, trimmed and thinly sliced into rounds
- 2 free-range eggs, beaten with a large pinch of salt
- 200g/7oz smoked mozzarella

Method

1 Preheat the oven to 200C/400F/Gas 6. Place the hollowed-out tomatoes onto kitchen paper. Add a pinch of salt, then turn the tomatoes over and set aside for 10-15 mins to drain of excess moisture.

2 Meanwhile, heat four tablespoons of the oil in a pan over a high heat. Add the onion and fry for 3-4 minutes, then add the reserved tomato pulp and half of the basil leaves, then season.

3 Reduce the heat to medium, cover and simmer for 20 mins, or until the moisture has evaporated and the mixture has thickened.

4 Heat 2 tbsp of olive oil in a separate frying pan over a medium heat. While the oil is heating, sprinkle the flour onto a plate and dredge the aubergine in the flour, shaking off any excess.

5 When the oil is hot, dip each aubergine round into the beaten egg. Add the coated aubergine to the hot oil, and fry for 3-4 minutes on each side, or until crisp and golden-brown on both sides. Season, to taste, with salt. Repeat the process with the remaining batches of aubergines, if necessary.

6 Add one fried aubergine slice to the cavity of each hollowed-out tomato, then top with a spoonful of the tomato sauce. Place a basil leaf on top of the sauce, then top with a slice of smoked mozzarella.

7 Repeat the process with all the tomatoes. Replace the 'lid' of each tomato and transfer to an ovenproof dish. Bake the stuffed tomatoes in the oven for 20 mins, or until the tomatoes have softened and the cheese has melted. To serve, garnish with basil leaves and drizzle over the remaining olive oil and season again.

CHICKEN TRAYBAKE

Ingredients

- 200g/7oz pack grilled artichokes
- 1½ tbsp olive oil
- 1 tsp dried oregano
- 2 tsp cumin seeds

- 8 chicken drumsticks
- 1 butternut squash, cut into chunks
- 150g/5oz roughly chopped mixed olives
- Large handful rocket

Method

1 Heat oven to 220C/425F/gas 6.

2 Measure out 1½ tbsp of oil from the grilled artichokes. Mix this with the olive oil, oregano and cumin. Put the chicken drumsticks and squash in a large roasting tin, toss in the flavoured oil and some seasoning.

3 Roast in the oven for 45 mins until tender and golden, then tip the artichokes and olives into the pan. Give everything a good mix, then return to the oven for 5 mins to warm through. Stir through the rocket and serve.

CHEF'S NOTE
This easy to make, one pan dish is low GI and paleo friendly. It's worth cooking more than you need for dinner, as the leftovers make a perfect lunch the next day.

CHICKEN AND QUINOA

Ingredients

- 1 tbsp cold-pressed rapeseed oil
- 2 skinless chicken breasts (about 300g/11oz)
- 100g/3½oz uncooked quinoa
- 1 medium onion, sliced into 12 wedges
- 1 red pepper, deseeded and sliced
- 2 garlic cloves, finely chopped
- 100g/3½oz green beans, trimmed and cut in half
- ¼-½ tsp chilli flakes, according to taste
- 2 tsp ground cumin
- 2 tsp ground coriander
- 75g/3oz frozen sweetcorn
- 75g/3oz kale, thickly shredded

Method

1 Heat the oil in a large, deep frying or sauté pan. Season the chicken and fry over a medium-high heat for 2-3 mins each side or until golden. Transfer to a plate. Add the onion and pepper to the pan and cook for 3 mins, stirring until softened and lightly browned.

2 Tip in the garlic and beans, and stir-fry for 2 mins. Add the chilli and spices, then stir in the quinoa and sweetcorn. Pour in 700ml just-boiled water with 1/2 tsp flaked sea salt and bring to the boil.

3 Return the chicken to the pan, reduce the heat to a simmer and cook for 12 mins, stirring regularly and turning the chicken occasionally. Add the kale and cook for a further 3 mins or until the quinoa and chicken are cooked through.

CHEF'S NOTE

Quinoa is a healthy grain that is high in protein, dietary fibre and B vitamins. Try it in place of rice or potatoes.

CURRIED COD

Ingredients

- 1 tbsp oil
- 1 onion, chopped
- 2 tbsp medium curry powder
- Thumb-sized piece ginger, peeled and finely grated
- 3 garlic cloves, crushed

- 400g/14oz tinned of chopped tomatoes
- 200g/7oz tinned of chickpeas
- 2 cod fillets (about 125-150g each)
- Zest 1 lemon, then cut into wedges
- Handful coriander, roughly chopped

Method

1 Heat the oil in a large, lidded frying pan. Cook the onion over a high heat for a few mins, then stir in the curry powder, ginger and garlic. Cook for another 1-2 mins until fragrant, then stir in the tomatoes, chickpeas and some seasoning.

2 Cook for 8-10 mins until thickened slightly, then top with the cod. Cover and cook for another 5-10 mins until the fish is cooked through.

3 Scatter over the lemon zest and coriander, then serve with the lemon wedges to squeeze over.

CHEF'S NOTE

Quick healthy and tasty, this one-pot meal dish is perfect for a midweek dinner and is bursting with protein and nutrients.

STUFFED PEPPERS

Ingredients

- 4 red peppers
- 1 courgette, quartered lengthways and thinly sliced
- 2 x 250g/9oz ready-to-eat quinoa
- 85g/3¼oz feta cheese, finely crumbled
- A handful of parsley, roughly chopped

Method

1 Heat oven to 200C/400F/gas 6. Cut each pepper in half through the stem, and remove the seeds. Put the peppers, cut-side up, on a baking sheet, drizzle with 1 tbsp olive oil and season well. Roast for 15 mins.

2 Meanwhile, heat 1 tsp olive oil in a small frying pan, add the courgette and cook until soft. Remove from the heat, then stir through the quinoa, feta and parsley. Season with pepper.

3 Divide the quinoa mixture between the pepper halves, then return to the oven for 5 mins to heat through.

CHEF'S NOTE
These stuffed peppers make a great side dish, or can also be served as the star of the show, with a dressed salad on the side.

DESSERT & SNACK
RECIPES

FRUIT FONDUE

Ingredients

- 300g/11oz mixed fruits; strawberries, pineapple chunks, grapes, mango chunks, melon chunks

- 150g/5oz of your favourite yoghurt
- 100g/3½oz dark chocolate

Method

1 Thread the fruits onto wooden skewers. Melt the chocolate on a low heat in the microwave or over a pan of boiling water and transfer to a small serving bowl.

2 Serve the kebabs on a platter with the yogurt and melted chocolate for dipping then get everyone to dig in.

CHEF'S NOTE
Although milk chocolate may be out of bounds, dark chocolate is low in sugar and high in iron, a mineral that plays an important part in thyroid hormone production.

TURKISH DELIGHT MESS

Ingredients

- 100g/3½oz mascarpone
- 50g/2oz Greek yogurt
- 25g/1oz sifted icing sugar
- 2 tbsp orange flower water
- 1 meringue nest, broken into rough pieces
- 3 apricots, stoned and chopped
- 2 cubes chopped diabetic Turkish delight, orange flavoured if available
- 25g/1oz skin-on almonds, roughly chopped

Method

1 Place the mascarpone, yogurt, sugar and orange flower water into a large bowl and whisk until thickened.

2 Fold the remaining ingredients through, then divide the mix between 2 dessert glasses or bowls.

CHEF'S NOTE

This dessert may taste exotic but it takes barely minutes to assemble. As refined sugar is off the menu it may be worth looking at diabetic sweets if you have a sweet tooth.

FRUITY YOGHURT JELLIES

Ingredients

- 4 sheets leaf gelatine
- 6 tbsp sugar-free lemon or orange squash
- ½ lemon, zest only, finely grated
- 150g/5oz fat-free natural yoghurt

- 200g/7oz mixed fresh berries (fresh or frozen)
- Small handful fresh mint leaves

Method

1 Put the gelatine sheets in a medium bowl and cover with cold water. Leave to soak for five minutes, or until they soften. Turn them a couple of times to make sure they don't stick together.

2 Pour the squash, lemon zest and 100ml/3½fl oz of water into a small saucepan and heat very gently until just warm. Remove from the heat.

3 Squeeze the gelatine sheets to remove excess water and then add to the pan, stirring until it melts in to the liquid.

4 Stir in 250ml/9fl oz water and the yoghurt until they are thoroughly combined.

5 Pour the jelly into four glass tumblers or dishes, cover with cling film and chill for 5-6 hours, or overnight, until set.

6 Serve the jellies topped with fresh berries and mint leaves to decorate.

CHEF'S NOTE
Using sugar free squash is a great way to inject fruity flavours with no refined sugar. Experiment with different juices to find your favourite flavour.

CARROT AND CHICK PEA TRAY BAKE

Ingredients

- 400g/14oz tin chickpeas, drained and rinsed
- 75g/3oz dates
- 1 tbsp vanilla extract
- 1 tbsp ground cinnamon
- ½ tsp bicarbonate of soda
- 1 free-range egg
- 3 pinches salt
- 1 tsp finely grated root ginger
- 1 large carrot, grated

Method

1 Preheat the oven to 180C/350F/Gas 4. Line a high-sided baking tray with baking parchment.

2 Blend all of the ingredients except the carrot in a food processor until smooth and well combined.

3 Add the carrot to the food processor and pulse a few times to combine, being careful not to over-blend.

4 Transfer the mixture to the prepared baking tray, spreading and smoothing it into an even layer using a palette knife.

5 Bake in the oven for 30-35 minutes, or until cooked through and browned on top. Remove and set aside to cool slightly, then cut into squares. Serve warm or cold.

CHEF'S NOTE

The ingredients may seem a little odd but the taste is more familiar, like carrot cake. The dates provide a natural sweetness and this would be perfect for an office or school cake sale.

FROZEN FRUIT STICKS WITH ZESTY SAUCE

Ingredients

- 100g/3½oz strawberries, hulled and halved
- 8 seedless grapes
- 125g/4oz mango chunks
- 125g/4oz melon chunks
- 2 kiwi fruit, peeled and cut into chunks
- 125g/4oz pineapple chunks
- For the sauce:
- Juice of 2 limes
- 4 passion fruits, halved and seeds scraped out

Method

1 Mix the sauce ingredients in a small bowl. If you want the sauce to be smooth, pass it through a sieve to remove the seeds, or leave them in if you prefer.

2 Skewer the fruits onto wooden skewers and drizzle the sauce on top, reserving a little for dipping.

3 Pop the skewers in the freezer for 45 mins, until just starting to freeze. Serve with the leftover sauce.

CHEF'S NOTE
Ice cream and lollies are something that may be hard to enjoy, but this frozen fruit has a tangy sweetness that's like a sorbet and hits the spot on a summer's day.

INSTANT ICE CREAM

Ingredients

- 250g/9oz frozen mixed berries
- 250g/9oz 0%-fat Greek yogurt
- 1 tbsp honey or agave syrup

Method

1 Blend the berries, yogurt and honey or agave syrup in a food processor for 20 seconds, until it comes together to a smooth ice-cream texture.

2 Scoop into bowls and serve.

CHEF'S NOTE
Keep the ingredients to hand for this and when cravings hit, you'll have all of the makings for a delicious fruity ice cream in seconds.

TROPICAL CREAMS

Ingredients

- 1 x 50g/2oz coconut cream
- 500g/1lb 2 oz Greek yogurt or quark
- A few drops vanilla extract
- 2 tsp honey
- 2 kiwi fruit
- 400g/14oz tinned pineapple chunks

Method

1 Dissolve the coconut cream in 50ml boiling water, then leave to cool. Spoon the quark or yogurt into a mixing bowl, then stir in the honey and vanilla. Combine with the coconut mix, then spoon into individual glasses. Chill until ready to serve.

2 Peel and chop the kiwi fruit into small pieces. Drain the pineapple, then chop the chunks into small pieces. Mix the fruit together, then spoon over the top of the coconut creams to serve.

CHEF'S NOTE

This tropical cream has all of the tastes of a piña colada but with none of the refined sugar. The natural sweetness from the fruit and honey make this a suitable treat.

MANGO AND LIME MOUSSE

Ingredients

- 2 sheets leaf gelatine
- 1 large ripe mango (approximately 450g/1lb)
- 1 lime, finely grated zest only
- 150ml/5fl oz double cream

Method

1 Half fill a bowl with cold water and add the gelatine sheets one at a time. Leave to soak for 5 minutes.

2 Cut the mango in half on either side of the large flat stone. Using a large spoon, scoop out the flesh and put into a food processor. Add the lime zest and blend until as smooth as possible.

3 Put 5 tablespoons of water in a small saucepan and heat very gently until lukewarm. Lift the gelatine sheets out of the cold water with your fingers and carefully drop into the warm water. Stir vigorously with a wooden spoon for a few seconds until the gelatine dissolves. Remove from the heat.

4 Whip the cream using an electric whisk in a large bowl until it stands in fairly stiff peaks.

5 With the motor running on the food processor, pour the gelatine solution slowly onto the mango purée and pulse until completely combined.

6 Put 6 tablespoons of the mango purée in a small bowl. Add the remaining purée to the whipped cream and whisk together lightly until smooth.

7 Spoon half the mango cream into four glass tumblers and spoon half the mango purée on top. Spoon the rest of the mango cream on top then finish with the remaining purée. Cover the dishes with cling film and chill for at least 3 hours before serving.

SPICED ORANGES

Ingredients

- 2 x 150g/5oz natural yoghurt
- 3 oranges
- Good pinch ground cinnamon
- 2 star anise

- ¼ tsp vanilla extract
- 1 tbsp unsalted pistachio nuts, roughly chopped (alternatively use toasted flaked almonds)

Method

1 Cut one of the oranges in half and squeeze out all the juice – you should end up with 4-5 tbsp. Peel the remaining oranges and cut into thin slices.

2 Pour the juice into a small saucepan and stir in the cinnamon, star anise and vanilla extract.

3 Place over a medium heat and simmer for 1-2 minutes, stirring occasionally. Add the orange slices and warm through gently.

4 Place the warm spiced oranges and juice into 2 bowls and spoon the yoghurt and scatter the nuts on top.

CHEF'S NOTE

This dessert has no refined sugar but harnesses the natural sweetness of the oranges, which is heightened by the heat, revealing their juicy sweetness.

BLUEBERRY RICOTTA POTS

Ingredients

- 200g/7oz ricotta
- Pinch ground cinnamon
- 2 tsp runny honey
- 200g/7oz blueberries

Method

1 Mix the ricotta with the cinnamon and half the honey in a bowl.

2 Gently stir in most of the blueberries. Divide the mixture between two ramekins or small bowls.

3 Top with the remaining blueberries and keep in the fridge, covered, until ready to eat.

4 Drizzle over the remaining honey just before serving.

CHEF'S NOTE
You may be more likely to encounter ricotta as part of a savoury meal, but much like mascarpone, this creamy cheese works perfectly when combined with sweet flavours.

CHOCOLATE ORANGE STEAMED PUDDING

Ingredients

For the chocolate sauce:
- 50g/2oz cocoa
- 50g/2oz butter, plus extra for greasing
- 100g/3½oz xylitol
- 1 tsp vanilla extract

- 200ml/7fl oz semi-skimmed milk

For the pudding:
- 1 small orange
- 100g/3½oz xylitol
- 225g/8oz self-raising flour
- 50g/2oz cocoa

- 150ml/5fl oz semi-skimmed milk
- 1 tsp vanilla extract
- 2 large eggs

Method

1 Begin by making the sauce. Sift the cocoa into a small saucepan, add all the other ingredients, then warm over a medium-high heat for 1 min to make a glossy sauce. Spoon 4 tbsp into the base of a lightly buttered, traditional 1.2 litre pudding basin. Leave the rest to cool, stirring occasionally.

2 Put a very large pan (deep enough to enclose the whole pudding basin) of water on to boil with a small upturned plate placed in the base.

3 Zest the orange, then cut the peel and pith away, and cut between the membrane to release the segments. Put all the pudding ingredients in a food processor and blitz.

4 Spoon the mixture into the pudding basin, smoothing to the edges.

5 Tear off a sheet of foil and a sheet of baking parchment, both about 30cm long. Butter the baking parchment and use to cover the foil. Fold a 3cm pleat in the middle of the sheets, then place over the pudding, buttered baking parchment-side down. Tie with string under the lip of the basin, making a handle as you go. Trim the excess parchment and foil to about 5cm, then tuck the foil around the parchment to seal. Lower the basin into the pan of water, checking that the water comes two-thirds of the way up the sides of the basin, then cover the pan with a lid to trap the steam and simmer for 90 mins.

6 Carefully unwrap the pudding – it should now be risen and firm – and turn out of the basin on to a plate. Spoon over some warmed sauce and serve the rest separately with slices of the pudding.

PINEAPPLE CHEESECAKE

Ingredients

For the base:
- 40g/1½oz butter
- 100g/3½oz oatcakes, crushed to crumbs
- 25g/1oz toasted desiccated coconut

For the topping
- 150g/5oz can coconut cream

- 425g/15oz tinned of pineapple in natural juice, drained
- 5 sheets of leaf gelatine
- 250g/9oz mascarpone
- 500g/1lb 2oz fromage frais
- Grated zest ½ lemon

Method

1 Melt the butter in a pan and stir in the oatcake crumbs and all but 1 tbsp of the desiccated coconut. Mix well then press very firmly onto the base of a lightly oiled 21cm spring-form tin to make a firm layer. Chill.

2 Finely chop a slice of pineapple then pulse the remainder to a pulp in a food processor, or with a hand blender. Soak the gelatine in cold water to soften it. In a bowl, beat together the mascarpone and fromage frais.

3 Very gently warm the coconut cream in a small pan. Squeeze the excess moisture from the gelatine, add to the warm coconut and stir until melted. Stir into the mascarpone mixture with the crushed and chopped pineapple and lemon zest then pour onto the biscuit base and chill until set.

4 Carefully remove from the tin, slide onto a plate, and decorate with the reserved coconut round the edge.

CHEF'S NOTE

This indulgent desert is kept low sugar by substituting the traditional biscuit base for one made with crushed oat biscuits and desiccated coconut.

PEANUT BUTTER BROWNIES

Ingredients

- 1 tsp vegetable oil, for greasing
- 500g/1lb 2oz dark chocolate, broken into pieces
- 3 large free-range eggs, at room temperature

- 1 tsp vanilla extract
- 165g/5¾oz good-quality crunchy peanut butter
- 180g/6oz ground almonds

Method

1 Preheat the oven to 180C/350F/Gas 4. Grease a 20cm/8in square tin with the oil and line with baking paper.

2 Melt the chocolate in a heatproof bowl set over a saucepan of gently simmering water.

3 Beat the eggs in a small bowl. Add them to the melted chocolate along with the vanilla extract and half the peanut butter. Mix together well.

4 Add the ground almonds to the mixture and stir in gently.

5 Pour the mixture into the prepared tin and level the surface. Drop spoonfuls of the remaining peanut butter over the top, creating swirls across the top of the mixture.

6 Bake in the preheated oven for 20 minutes, or until cracks appear on the surface.

7 Leave to cool in in the tin. Remove, cut into 9 brownie squares and serve.

CHEF'S NOTE

Dark, damp and delicious, these brownies are exactly what you want from a dessert. Perhaps surprisingly, they contain no sugar and are gluten free.

COCONUT MACAROONS

Ingredients

- 80g/2¾oz desiccated coconut
- 125ml/4½fl oz full-fat coconut milk
- 1 tbsp coconut flour

- 2 tbsp maple syrup
- ½ tsp vanilla extract
- A pinch of salt

Method

1 Preheat the oven to 180C/350F/Gas 4. Line a baking tray with baking parchment.

2 Stir all of the ingredients together in a saucepan over a medium heat until well combined. Continue to cook for 4-5 minutes until the coconut milk has been absorbed and the mixture has thickened. Remove from the heat and set aside to cool slightly.

3 Scoop tablespoonful's of the macaroon mixture onto the prepared baking tray, to form small domes, leaving a gap between each. Bake in the middle of the oven for 12-15 minutes, or until toasted and golden brown at the edges.

4 Remove from the oven and set the macaroons aside to cool completely, then enjoy.

CHEF'S NOTE

These deliciously moist macaroons contain lots of healthy fats from the coconut milk and are perfect for an after dinner or mid-afternoon treat.

BAKED APPLES

Ingredients

- 4 cooking apples, cored but left whole
- 2 stem ginger balls, finely chopped
- ½ tsp ground cinnamon
- 4 prunes, chopped
- 50g/2oz light muscovado sugar
- 1 tbsp butter

Method

1 Heat your oven to 200C/400F/gas 6. Using a sharp knife, score a line around the centre of each apple. Put them into a baking dish with a small splash of water in the bottom.

2 In a bowl, combine the ginger, cinnamon, prunes and sugar. Stuff the mixture into the apples so that they are well packed. Top each with a knob of butter and bake for 35-40 mins, or until cooked through. To test, pierce with a sharp knife – it should slide straight through.

3 Remove from the oven and baste the apples with the liquid left in the dish. Serve hot or warm with cream or yoghurt.

4 The apples can be cooked up to a day ahead, then warmed through in the oven or microwave before eating.

CHEF'S NOTE

Baked apples are a delicious autumnal dish, that has all of the flavours of apple pie but no gluten and is far less work!

BUCKS FIZZ JELLIES

Ingredients

- 7 sheets gelatine
- 600ml/1pt orange juice
- 300ml/10½fl oz prosecco

Method

1 Put the gelatine sheets into a bowl of cold water to soften for a few mins. Put 100ml of clementine juice into a small pan and gently heat. When the gelatine feels soft and the juice is just simmering, remove the juice from the heat and squeeze out any excess water from the gelatine sheets. Drop the sheets into the hot juice and swirl to melt. Make sure there are no visible lumps of gelatine before you move onto the next stage.

2 Stir the hot juice into the remaining juice with the prosecco, then transfer to a jug. Pour between 6 small glasses. Sit the jellies in a small tray or dish, cover with a sheet of cling film and chill for at least 4 hrs (or up to 48 hrs) until set.

CHEF'S NOTE

This is the perfect make ahead dessert for if you're entertaining. The combination of prosecco and orange juice makes this a festive treat.

COCONUT BLONDIES

Ingredients

- 100g/3½oz ground almonds
- 2 tbsp coconut flour
- 40g/1½oz coconut sugar
- Pinch baking soda
- 1 tbsp ground flaxseeds
- 3 tbsp water

- 1 tbsp almond butter
- 2 tsp melted coconut oil
- 1 tsp vanilla extract
- 3 tbsp dark chocolate chips
- 2 tbsp roasted pistachios

Method

1 Preheat the oven to 170C/325F/Gas 3 and line the bottom of a 4×7-inch baking dish with parchment paper.

2 In a small bowl, whisk together the ground flaxseeds with the 3 tablespoons of water and eggs and let it sit for 5 minutes. It should become thick and viscous.

3 In a large mixing bowl, whisk together the almond flour, coconut flour, coconut sugar and baking soda. Add the flax seed and egg mixture, almond butter, coconut oil and vanilla extract. Mix using a spoon or spatula until combined. It should have the texture of cookie dough.

4 Stir in the dark chocolate chips and roasted pistachios, then mix again until combined.

5 Transfer the dough to the prepared pan and press it down into an even layer. You can use a layer of parchment paper and a glass to press it down if the dough is too sticky.

6 Bake for 10-12 minutes, or until the top of the blondies is slightly golden brown.

7 Remove from the oven and let it cool completely before cutting into small squares. Blondies will keep at room temperature in an airtight container for up to 5 days.

CHEF'S NOTE
You can find coconut flour in many larger supermarkets or it's easy to source online.

KALE, PEA AND RICOTTA FRITTERS

Ingredients

- 125g/4oz frozen peas, thawed and crushed
- 150g/5oz kale leaves, finely shredded
- 250g/9oz fresh ricotta
- 3 free-range eggs

- 50g/2oz chia seeds
- 1 tbsp lemon zest (approx. 1 lemon)
- 2 tbsp chopped fresh mint
- 2 tbsp extra virgin olive oil

Method

1 Put all the ingredients, except the oil, in a bowl and mix. Season with salt and pepper and set aside for 20 minutes.

2 To cook the fritters, heat a little oil in a large frying pan over a medium heat. Take about 2 tablespoons of the mixture and shape into a patty, flatten slightly. Cook in batches for 2–3 minutes on each side until golden brown, adding more oil if necessary.

3 Divide the fritters between serving plates.

CHEF'S NOTE

These vegetarian fritters are bursting with goodness and make a wonderful snack or starter when accompanied by a salad and lemon wedges.

CHICKEN SKEWERS

Ingredients

- 4 chicken mini-fillets
- 1 tbsp soy sauce
- 1 orange, zest only

- 2 tbsp olive oil
- 8 mini wooden skewers, soaked in water for ten minutes

Method

1 Slice each mini-fillet in half lengthways and place in a small bowl and add the soy sauce, orange zest and olive oil. Leave to marinade for 5 mins.

2 Thread each chicken mini-fillet onto a skewer. Heat a griddle pan and fry the chicken skewers for 3 mins on each side, or until cooked through. Serve immediately.

CHEF'S NOTE

These protein packed mini skewers are perfect for either an afternoon snack, or as a dinner party starter when accompanied by some salad garnish.

SMOKED FISH OATCAKES

Ingredients

- ½ Arbroath smokie or smoked salmon fillet skinned, boned and flaked into small pieces
- 2 tbsp Greek yoghurt
- 1 tbsp chopped fresh dill
- 1 tbsp chopped fresh chives
- Juice of ½ lemon
- 6 small oatcakes
- 6 thin slices of cucumber
- ½ ripe tomato, chopped and seeds removed

Method

1 First make the pâté by placing the fish, yoghurt and herbs into a bowl and mash together with a fork.

2 Spread some of the pâté onto each of the oatcakes and top with the cucumber, chopped tomato and a drop of lemon juice.

CHEF'S NOTE

A good source of iodine, selenium and zinc these oatcakes are adaptable. Serve as a starter, snack or even a party canapé.

QUINOA AND POMEGRANATE SALAD

Ingredients

- 300g/11oz quinoa
- 1 red onion, finely chopped
- 85g/3¼oz raisins or sultanas
- 100g/3½oz feta cheese, crumbled
- 200g/7oz pomegranate seeds

- 85g/3¼oz toasted flaked almonds
- Small pack each coriander, flat leaf parsley and mint, roughly chopped
- Juice of 3 lemons

Method

1 Cook the quinoa following pack instructions – it should be tender but with a little bite. Drain well and spread over a platter or wide, shallow bowl to cool quickly and steam dry.

2 When the quinoa is just about cool stir through all of the remaining ingredients with plenty of seasoning.

CHEF'S NOTE

This low GI dish is an excellent accompaniment to meat or fish. If you have any leftovers then mix through the meat or fish and you'll have a tasty lunch.

BUTTER BEAN SALAD

Ingredients

- 540g/1lb 3oz jar large butter beans
- 500g/1lb 2oz tomatoes, peeled and cored
- 1 red chilli
- A bunch of basil
- 1 garlic clove
- 1 tbsp olive oil
- 1 tbsp red wine vinegar

Method

1 Drain and rinse the butter beans and place in a mixing bowl. Chop the tomatoes and add to the beans.

2 Place the chilli, basil (reserving a few small leaves) garlic, olive oil and vinegar in the small bowl of a food processor, then whizz until smooth.

3 Add to the tomatoes and beans, season and mix. Serve scattered with a few small leaves.

CHEF'S NOTE

This salad is super-healthy and contains 2 of your 5 a day! You can warm the beans and tomato before adding the sauce for a different version during cooler months.

SPICED CAULIFLOWER AND CHICKPEAS

Ingredients

- 1 large head of cauliflower, broken into florets
- 2 garlic cloves, crushed
- 2 tsp each caraway and cumin seeds
- 3 tbsp olive oil
- 400g/14oz tin of chickpeas, drained and rinsed
- 100g/3½oz pine nuts
- Small bunch each parsley and dill, leaves torn

Method

1 Heat oven to 200C/400f/gas 6. Toss the cauliflower, garlic, spices, 2 tbsp oil and some seasoning in a roasting tin, and then roast for 30 mins.

2 Add the chickpeas, pine nuts and remaining oil to the tin, then cook for 10 mins more. To serve, stir in the herbs.

CHEF'S NOTE
Cauliflower is perhaps one of the most adaptable vegetables for you to eat if you're limiting your grain consumption. Try making cauliflower rice or mash.

FRUIT AND NUT BARS

Ingredients

- 400g/14oz soft pitted dates
- 300g/10½oz cashew nut pieces
- 4 tbsp cacao or cocoa powder
- 1 tbsp almond butter
- 1 tbsp coconut oil
- 1 tbsp vanilla essence

Method

1 Grease and line a 20x20cm/8x8in baking tray. Put all the ingredients into a food processor and blend until the cashew nuts become tiny pieces.

2 Remove the lid and add 1 tablespoon of water and blend again. If the mixture is not already sticking together, add another spoon of water and blend again. Repeat until the mixture starts to stick together.

3 Using a spoonful or spatula, transfer the mixture into the lined tray. Press the mixture into the tray and put in the fridge to set for at least an hour.

4 Remove from the fridge and slice into 12 bars or smaller chunks. Wrap individually in greaseproof paper and keep in the fridge until you need a healthy snack on the go.

CHEF'S NOTE

When you hear a chocolate bar calling to you, indulge in one of these instead. The cocoa, nuts and sweet dates will make sure your sweet tooth is left satisfied.

TUNA PROTEIN POT

Ingredients

- 1 large egg
- 80g/3oz green beans
- 1 tomato
- 120g/4oz can tuna in spring water
- 1½ -2 tbsp French dressing

Method

1 Boil the egg for 8 mins and steam the green beans for 6 mins above the pan until tender.

2 Cool the egg and beans under running water then carefully peel and quarter the egg. Leave to cool.

3 Tip the beans into a large packed lunch pot. Top with the tomato, tuna and quartered egg and spoon on the French dressing. Seal until ready to eat.

CHEF'S NOTE

This protein pot has all of the flavours you'd find in a niçoise salad but with much less fuss. Packed full of selenium, this is a perfect snack for a healthy thyroid.

KALE CRISPS

Ingredients

- ½ tsp dried chilli flakes
- 1 tsp garlic granules
- ¼ tsp sea salt
- 250g/9oz curly kale, leaves picked from stems, washed and dried
- 1 tbsp light olive oil

Method

1 Preheat the oven to 120C/250F Fan/Gas ½ and line two large baking trays with baking paper.

2 Mix together the chilli, garlic granules and sea salt.

3 Put the kale in a large bowl and massage the oil into the leaves. Toss with the seasoning.

4 Spread the leaves out in a single layer on the baking trays. Bake for 20 minutes, turning the trays halfway through cooking.

5 Lift the leaves from the baking paper using a spatula. Return the trays to the oven, turn off the heat and leave for 12–15 minutes, or until crisp.

CHEF'S NOTE

When the urge to eat something crisp and salty hits, these kale crisps are the perfect substitute for potato crisps.

FRUIT TRUFFLES

Ingredients

- 50g/2oz soft dried apricot
- 100g/4oz soft dried date
- 50g/2oz dried cherry

- 2 tsp coconut oil
- 1 tbsp toasted sesame seeds

Method

1 Blitz the apricots with the dates and cherries in a food processor until very finely chopped. Tip into a bowl and use your hands to work in the coconut oil.

2 Shape the mix into walnut-sized balls, then roll in sesame seeds. Store in an airtight container.

CHEF'S NOTE
The perfect snack for when you need a quick energy fix. These fruity bites are paleo friendly and gluten free.

LEMON COOKIES

Ingredients

- 150g/5oz ground almonds
- 1 tbsp arrowroot
- ¼ tsp salt
- ¼ tsp bicarbonate of soda
- 2 tbsp maple syrup
- ½ tsp fresh thyme or lemon-thyme leaves, or to taste
- 1 tbsp grated lemon zest

Method

1 Preheat the oven to 180C/350F/Gas 4. Line a baking tray with baking parchment.

2 Pulse the almonds, arrowroot, salt and bicarbonate of soda in a food processor until the mixture is well combined and resembles breadcrumbs.

3 Add the maple syrup, thyme leaves and lemon zest and pulse again until the mixture comes together as a ball of dough.

4 Remove the dough from the food processor. Tear off 10 equal-sized pieces of the dough and roll them into golf-ball-sized balls, then flatten each between the palms of your hands and place onto the prepared baking tray, leaving plenty of space between each cookie.

5 Bake for 10-12 minutes, or until crisp and golden brown at the edges. Remove the tray from the oven and set aside to cool. The cookies will crisp up as they cool, but will still be soft in the middle.

CHEF'S NOTE

These squidgy biscuits are bursting with zesty flavour and perfect for an afternoon snack when the cookie jar is calling you!

LEMON HUMMUS

Ingredients

- 2 x 400g/14oz tinned chickpeas in water, drained
- 2 fat garlic cloves, roughly chopped
- 3 tbsp Greek yogurt
- 3 tbsp tahini paste
- 3 tbsp extra-virgin olive oil, plus extra
- Zest and juice of 2 lemons
- Handful of fresh coriander

Method

1 Put everything but the coriander into a food processor, then whizz to a fairly smooth mix. Scrape down the sides of the processor if you need to.

2 Season the hummus generously, then add the coriander and pulse until roughly chopped. Spoon into a serving bowl, drizzle with olive oil, then serve.

CHEF'S NOTE

Hummus is full of zinc, protein and healthy fats, making it a perfect snack for filling you up. Serve with crudités of your choosing.

Made in the USA
Las Vegas, NV
24 February 2023

68035290R00057